This publication is intended to provide educational information for the reader on the covered subjects. It is not intended to take the place of personalized medical counseling, diagnosis, and treatment from a trained healthcare professional.

ISBN 978-1-998455-47-8 (Paperback)
ISBN 978-1-998455-48-5 (eBook)

Printed and bound in USA
Published by Loons Press

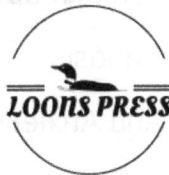

I0096766

LOONS PRESS

Table Of Contents

How To Recover From Leukemia Or Lymphoma

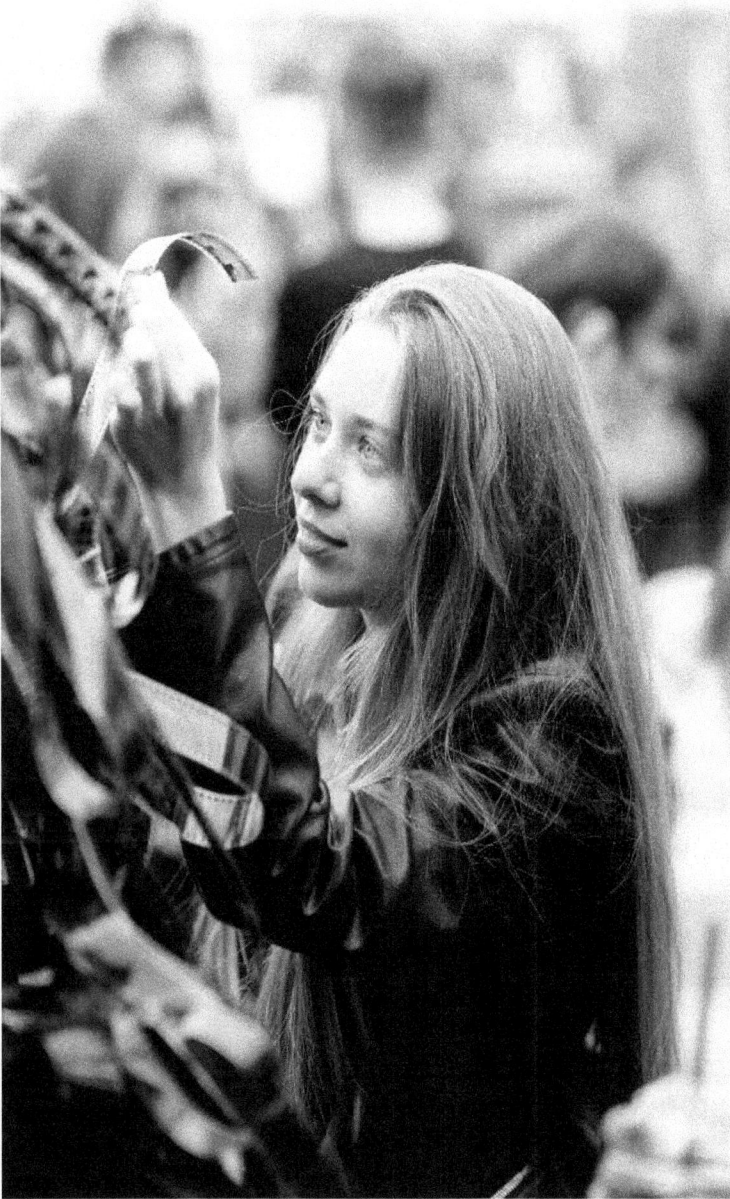

A Roadmap to Healing

Chapter 1

Understanding Leukemia and Lymphoma

What is Leukemia?

Leukemia is a type of cancer that affects the blood and bone marrow. It is characterized by the abnormal production of white blood cells, which are responsible for fighting off infections in the body. Leukemia can be classified into four main types: acute lymphoblastic leukemia (ALL), acute myeloid leukemia (AML), chronic lymphocytic leukemia (CLL), and chronic myeloid leukemia (CML). Each type of leukemia has its own unique characteristics and treatment options.

One of the key features of leukemia is the uncontrolled growth of white blood cells, which can crowd out healthy blood cells and lead to a variety of symptoms. These symptoms can include fatigue, weakness, frequent infections, easy bruising or bleeding, and weight loss.

The diagnosis of leukemia is typically made through a blood test or bone marrow biopsy, which can reveal the presence of abnormal cells.

Treatment for leukemia depends on the type and stage of the cancer, as well as the patient's overall health and preferences. Common treatment options include chemotherapy, radiation therapy, targeted therapy, and stem cell transplant. These treatments can help to destroy cancer cells, reduce symptoms, and improve quality of life.

Recovering from leukemia can be a long and challenging process, but with the right support and resources, it is possible to thrive after a diagnosis. It is important for patients to work closely with their healthcare team to develop a personalized treatment plan and to seek out additional support from family, friends, and support groups.

Making healthy lifestyle choices, such as eating a balanced diet, exercising regularly, and managing stress, can also help to improve overall well-being and recovery.

In conclusion, leukemia is a complex and challenging disease, but with the right knowledge and support, it is possible to recover and thrive after a diagnosis. By understanding the basics of leukemia, exploring treatment options, and making healthy lifestyle choices, patients can take control of their health and work towards a successful recovery. Remember, you are not alone in this journey – there are resources and support available to help you every step of the way.

Types of Leukemia

Leukemia is a type of cancer that affects the blood and bone marrow, causing an overproduction of abnormal white blood cells. There are several different types of leukemia, each with its own characteristics and treatment options.

Understanding the different types of leukemia is crucial for those who have been diagnosed with the disease, as it can help guide treatment decisions and provide insight into what to expect during the recovery process.

The most common types of leukemia are acute lymphoblastic leukemia (ALL), acute myeloid leukemia (AML), chronic lymphocytic leukemia (CLL), and chronic myeloid leukemia (CML). ALL and AML are classified as acute leukemias, which means they progress quickly and require immediate treatment. CLL and CML, on the other hand, are considered chronic leukemias, which progress more slowly and may not require treatment right away.

Acute lymphoblastic leukemia (ALL) is the most common type of leukemia in children, but it can also affect adults. It is characterized by the rapid proliferation of immature lymphocytes in the bone marrow and blood. Acute myeloid leukemia (AML), on the other hand, is characterized by the rapid proliferation of abnormal myeloid cells in the bone marrow and blood. AML is more common in adults than in children.

Chronic lymphocytic leukemia (CLL) is a slow-growing leukemia that affects a type of white blood cell called B lymphocytes. CLL is most commonly diagnosed in older adults and often progresses slowly, with some patients never requiring treatment.

Chronic myeloid leukemia (CML) is characterized by the overproduction of abnormal myeloid cells in the bone marrow and blood. CML progresses slowly at first but can transform into a more aggressive form if left untreated.

Understanding the different types of leukemia is essential for those who have been diagnosed with the disease. It can help patients and their loved ones make informed decisions about treatment options and provide insight into what to expect during the recovery process. By working closely with healthcare providers and staying informed about their specific type of leukemia, individuals can take an active role in their recovery and improve their overall quality of life.

What is Lymphoma?

Lymphoma is a type of cancer that affects the lymphatic system, which is a vital part of the immune system. The lymphatic system includes lymph nodes, spleen, thymus, and bone marrow, all of which play a critical role in fighting infections and diseases. Lymphoma occurs when abnormal lymphocytes, a type of white blood cell, grow out of control and form tumors in the lymph nodes or other parts of the body.

There are two main types of lymphoma: Hodgkin lymphoma and non-Hodgkin lymphoma. Hodgkin lymphoma is characterized by the presence of Reed-Sternberg cells, which are large, abnormal cells that are typically found in the lymph nodes. Non-Hodgkin lymphoma, on the other hand, encompasses a diverse group of lymphomas that do not contain Reed-Sternberg cells. Both types of lymphoma can be further classified into subtypes based on the specific type of cells involved and other factors.

Symptoms of lymphoma can vary depending on the type and stage of the disease, but common symptoms include swollen lymph nodes, fever, night sweats, unexplained weight loss, and fatigue. Diagnosing lymphoma typically involves a combination of physical exams, blood tests, imaging tests, and biopsies of affected lymph nodes or tissues. Treatment for lymphoma may include chemotherapy, radiation therapy, immunotherapy, targeted therapy, or stem cell transplant, depending on the type and stage of the disease.

Recovering from lymphoma can be a challenging process that requires physical, emotional, and mental strength. It is important for individuals with lymphoma to work closely with their healthcare team to develop a personalized treatment plan and to follow through with all recommended treatments and follow-up care.

Support from family, friends, and other survivors can also play a crucial role in the recovery process, providing encouragement, understanding, and a sense of community.

While the road to recovery from lymphoma may be long and difficult, it is possible to thrive after a diagnosis. By taking an active role in their treatment, staying informed about their condition, and maintaining a positive attitude, individuals with lymphoma can increase their chances of a successful recovery.

With the right support and resources, it is possible to not only survive lymphoma but to thrive and live a fulfilling life beyond cancer.

Types of Lymphoma

Lymphoma is a type of cancer that affects the lymphatic system, which is a vital part of the immune system. There are two main types of lymphoma: Hodgkin lymphoma and non-Hodgkin lymphoma. Hodgkin lymphoma is characterized by the presence of Reed-Sternberg cells, while non-Hodgkin lymphoma includes a wide variety of subtypes that can be further classified based on the cells involved and their characteristics.

One common subtype of non-Hodgkin lymphoma is diffuse large B-cell lymphoma (DLBCL), which is the most common type of non-Hodgkin lymphoma in adults. DLBCL is an aggressive form of lymphoma that requires prompt treatment.

Another subtype is follicular lymphoma, which is a slow-growing type of lymphoma that may not require immediate treatment. Other subtypes of non-Hodgkin lymphoma include mantle cell lymphoma, marginal zone lymphoma, and Burkitt lymphoma, among others.

On the other hand, Hodgkin lymphoma is characterized by the presence of Reed-Sternberg cells, which are large, abnormal cells that help distinguish this type of lymphoma from non-Hodgkin lymphoma. Hodgkin lymphoma is further classified into subtypes based on the characteristics of the Reed-Sternberg cells and other factors. The most common subtype of Hodgkin lymphoma is nodular sclerosis Hodgkin lymphoma, followed by mixed cellularity Hodgkin lymphoma, lymphocyte-rich Hodgkin lymphoma, and lymphocyte-depleted Hodgkin lymphoma.

It is important for individuals with leukemia or lymphoma to understand the different types of lymphoma, as each type may require a different treatment approach. Treatment options for lymphoma may include chemotherapy, radiation therapy, immunotherapy, targeted therapy, stem cell transplant, or a combination of these treatments. The choice of treatment will depend on the type and stage of the lymphoma, as well as the individual's overall health and preferences. It is essential for individuals with leukemia or lymphoma to work closely with their healthcare team to develop a personalized treatment plan that addresses their specific needs and goals.

In conclusion, there are several types of lymphoma, each with its own characteristics and treatment options. By understanding the different types of lymphoma and working closely with their healthcare team, individuals with leukemia or lymphoma can make informed decisions about their treatment and improve their chances of recovery. It is important for individuals with leukemia or lymphoma to stay informed, ask questions, and advocate for their health to thrive after diagnosis.

How To Recover From Leukemia Or Lymphoma

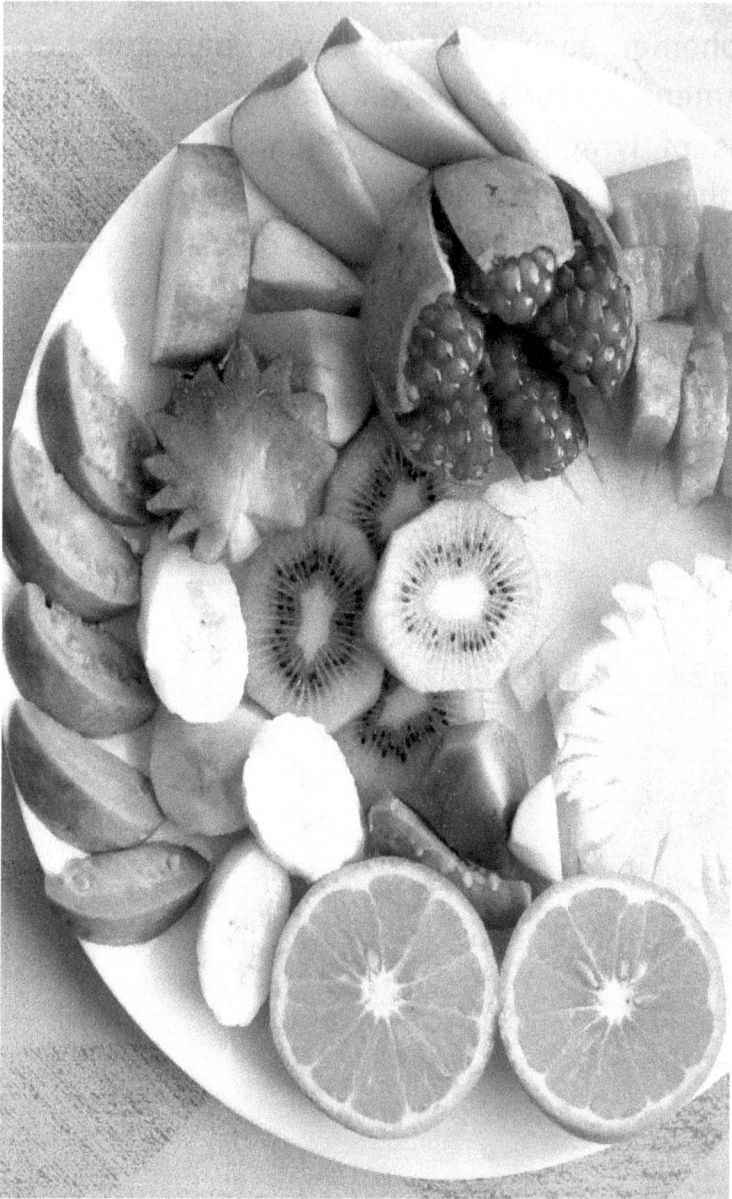

Chapter 2

Diagnosis and Treatment Options

Symptoms and Diagnosis

Symptoms of leukemia and lymphoma can vary depending on the type and stage of the cancer. Common symptoms of leukemia include fatigue, weakness, frequent infections, unexplained weight loss, and swollen lymph nodes. Additionally, individuals with leukemia may experience easy bruising, nosebleeds, and bone pain. On the other hand, symptoms of lymphoma may include swollen lymph nodes, fever, night sweats, unexplained weight loss, and fatigue.

It is important to note that these symptoms can be caused by other conditions as well, so it is crucial to consult with a healthcare provider for an accurate diagnosis.

Diagnosing leukemia and lymphoma typically involves a series of tests and procedures to confirm the presence of cancer. Blood tests, such as a complete blood count (CBC) and blood smear, can help identify abnormal levels of white blood cells, red blood cells, and platelets. Additionally, a bone marrow biopsy may be performed to examine the bone marrow for cancer cells. Imaging tests, such as CT scans and PET scans, can also help determine the extent of the cancer and whether it has spread to other parts of the body.

Once a diagnosis of leukemia or lymphoma is confirmed, it is important to work closely with a healthcare team to develop a treatment plan. Treatment options for leukemia and lymphoma may include chemotherapy, radiation therapy, targeted therapy, immunotherapy, or stem cell transplantation.

The goal of treatment is to eliminate cancer cells, prevent recurrence, and improve overall quality of life. It is important for individuals with leukemia or lymphoma to discuss all treatment options with their healthcare providers to determine the best course of action for their specific situation.

In addition to medical treatment, individuals with leukemia or lymphoma may benefit from complementary therapies to help manage symptoms and improve overall well-being. These may include acupuncture, massage therapy, yoga, meditation, and dietary supplements.

It is important to consult with a healthcare provider before incorporating any complementary therapies into a treatment plan to ensure they are safe and effective. By taking a holistic approach to care, individuals with leukemia or lymphoma can optimize their recovery and thrive after cancer.

Overall, understanding the symptoms and diagnosis process of leukemia and lymphoma is essential for individuals navigating their cancer journey. By recognizing common symptoms, seeking prompt medical attention, and actively participating in treatment decisions, individuals with leukemia or lymphoma can take control of their health and work towards healing and recovery. With the support of a healthcare team, loved ones, and a positive mindset, it is possible to thrive after leukemia and lymphoma.

Traditional Treatment Methods

When diagnosed with leukemia or lymphoma, it's crucial to explore all possible treatment options to ensure the best possible outcome. Traditional treatment methods have been used for decades to effectively combat these types of cancer.

These methods include chemotherapy, radiation therapy, and stem cell transplants. While these treatments can be challenging and come with potential side effects, they have been proven to be effective in fighting leukemia and lymphoma.

Chemotherapy is a common treatment method for leukemia and lymphoma, involving the use of powerful drugs to kill cancer cells. This treatment can be administered orally or intravenously and is often done in cycles to allow the body to recover in between treatments.

While chemotherapy can have side effects such as hair loss, nausea, and fatigue, it is a critical component in the fight against these types of cancer.

Radiation therapy is another traditional treatment method used for leukemia and lymphoma. This treatment involves the use of high-energy radiation beams to target and destroy cancer cells. Radiation therapy can be used alone or in combination with other treatments such as chemotherapy. While it can also have side effects such as skin irritation and fatigue, it is a highly effective method for treating these types of cancer.

Stem cell transplants are a more advanced traditional treatment method that can be used for certain types of leukemia and lymphoma. This procedure involves replacing damaged or diseased bone marrow with healthy stem cells to help the body produce new, healthy blood cells. While stem cell transplants can be a more intensive treatment with potential risks, they can also offer a chance for long-term remission and even a cure for some patients.

In conclusion, traditional treatment methods such as chemotherapy, radiation therapy, and stem cell transplants have been essential in the fight against leukemia and lymphoma.

While these treatments can be challenging and come with potential side effects, they have been proven to be effective in treating these types of cancer. It's important for individuals with leukemia or lymphoma to work closely with their healthcare team to explore all possible treatment options and make informed decisions about their care.

Alternative Treatment Approaches

When it comes to recovering from leukemia and lymphoma, exploring alternative treatment approaches can offer new avenues for healing and support. While traditional medical treatments like chemotherapy and radiation therapy are often the first line of defense against these cancers, alternative therapies can complement and enhance the healing process.

These approaches focus on treating the whole person - body, mind, and spirit - and can provide additional support in managing symptoms, reducing side effects, and promoting overall well-being.

One alternative treatment approach to consider is acupuncture. This ancient practice involves the insertion of thin needles into specific points on the body to promote healing and balance energy flow. Acupuncture has been shown to help alleviate pain, reduce nausea and fatigue, and improve overall quality of life for cancer patients.

By stimulating the body's natural healing mechanisms, acupuncture can support the immune system and enhance the body's ability to fight off cancer cells.

Another alternative therapy to explore is meditation and mindfulness. These practices involve focusing on the present moment, calming the mind, and cultivating a sense of inner peace and relaxation.

Studies have shown that meditation can reduce stress, anxiety, and depression in cancer patients, as well as improve overall quality of life. By incorporating meditation and mindfulness into your daily routine, you can create a sense of calm and balance that can support your healing journey.

Nutritional therapy is another alternative approach that can play a crucial role in recovering from leukemia and lymphoma. Eating a balanced diet rich in fruits, vegetables, whole grains, and lean proteins can help boost your immune system, reduce inflammation, and support overall health.

Working with a nutritionist or dietitian can help you create a personalized meal plan that meets your specific nutritional needs and supports your body's healing process.

In addition to these alternative treatment approaches, it's important to remember that each person's journey to recovery is unique. What works for one individual may not work for another, so it's important to explore different options and find what resonates with you.

By taking a holistic approach to healing and incorporating alternative therapies into your treatment plan, you can empower yourself to thrive after leukemia and lymphoma.

Managing Side Effects

Managing side effects is an essential aspect of the journey to recovery for individuals who have been diagnosed with leukemia or lymphoma. While undergoing treatment, it is common to experience a range of side effects that can impact your daily life. By learning how to effectively manage these side effects, you can improve your overall quality of life and increase your chances of a successful recovery.

One of the key strategies for managing side effects is to communicate openly with your healthcare team. Your doctors and nurses are there to support you and can provide valuable advice on how to cope with side effects such as nausea, fatigue, and pain. By sharing your symptoms and concerns with your healthcare team, they can tailor your treatment plan to better address your individual needs.

In addition to seeking guidance from your healthcare team, it is important to take a proactive approach to managing side effects. This may involve making lifestyle changes, such as adopting a healthy diet, staying physically active, and getting enough rest.

By taking care of your body and mind, you can help alleviate some of the side effects associated with leukemia or lymphoma treatment.

It is also crucial to seek support from friends, family, and other individuals who have gone through similar experiences. Talking to others who understand what you are going through can provide emotional support and practical advice on how to cope with side effects. Support groups and online communities can be valuable resources for connecting with others who are on a similar journey to recovery.

Ultimately, managing side effects is a continuous process that requires patience, perseverance, and self-care. By staying informed, communicating with your healthcare team, making lifestyle changes, and seeking support from others, you can effectively manage side effects and improve your overall well-being as you navigate the challenges of leukemia or lymphoma treatment. Remember, you are not alone in this journey, and there are resources available to help you thrive after leukemia or lymphoma.

How To Recover From Leukemia Or Lymphoma

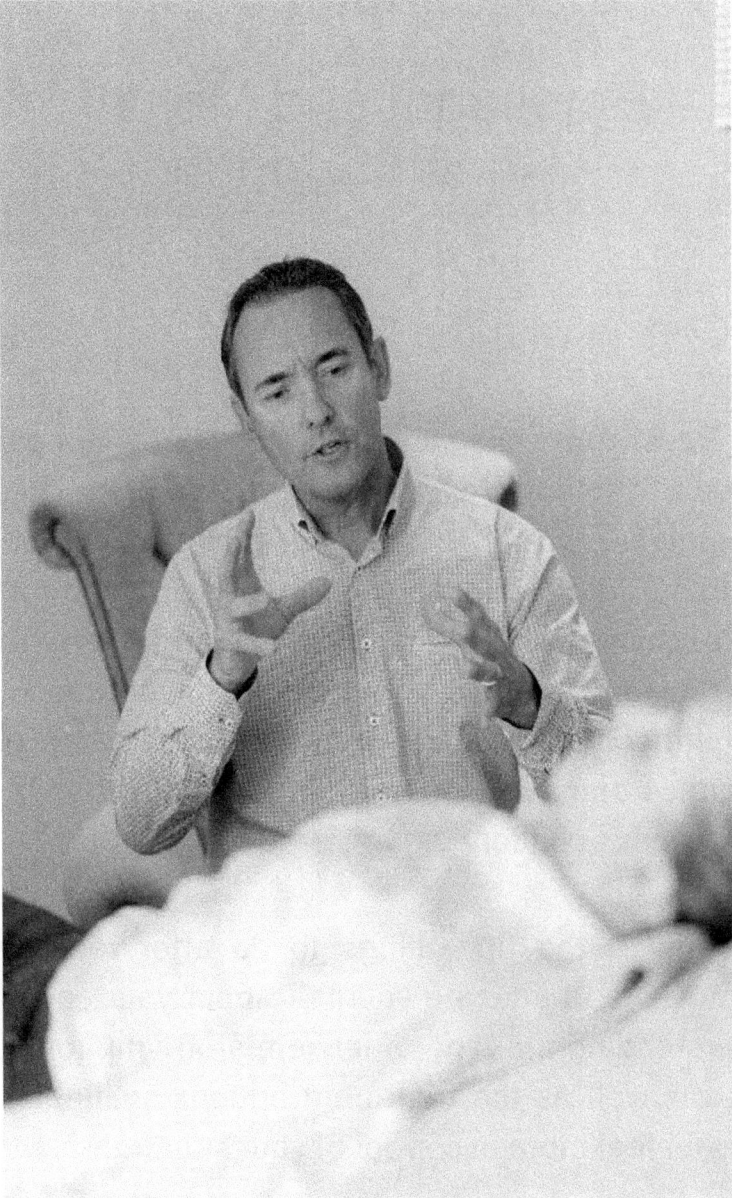

Chapter 3

Emotional and Mental Health Support

Coping with the Diagnosis

Receiving a diagnosis of leukemia or lymphoma can be a frightening and overwhelming experience. It is completely normal to feel a range of emotions, including fear, sadness, and uncertainty about the future. Coping with the diagnosis is an important first step in your journey towards healing and recovery. Remember that you are not alone - there are many resources and support systems available to help you navigate this challenging time.

One of the first things to do after receiving a diagnosis is to educate yourself about your condition. Understanding the type of leukemia or lymphoma you have, as well as the treatment options available, can help you feel more in control of your situation.

Ask your healthcare team any questions you may have and don't be afraid to seek out additional information from reputable sources. Knowledge is power, and arming yourself with information can help alleviate some of the anxiety surrounding your diagnosis.

It is also important to take care of your emotional well-being during this time. Coping with a serious illness can take a toll on your mental health, so be sure to prioritize self-care. This may include seeking support from friends and family, joining a support group for individuals with leukemia or lymphoma, or speaking with a mental health professional. Remember that it is okay to feel a range of emotions and that seeking help is a sign of strength, not weakness.

In addition to taking care of your emotional well-being, it is important to focus on your physical health as well. Eating a healthy diet, getting regular exercise, and getting plenty of rest can help support your body as it undergoes treatment for leukemia or lymphoma. Your healthcare team can provide you with guidance on how to best care for yourself during this time, so don't hesitate to ask for their advice.

Finally, remember that recovery from leukemia or lymphoma is possible. While the road ahead may be long and challenging, many individuals have successfully overcome these diseases and gone on to live full, healthy lives.

Stay positive, stay connected to your support system, and trust in your healthcare team to guide you through this difficult time. You are stronger than you think, and with the right mindset and support, you can thrive after leukemia or lymphoma.

Dealing with Fear and Anxiety

Fear and anxiety are common emotions that can arise during and after a battle with leukemia or lymphoma. It is important to acknowledge these feelings and address them in a healthy way in order to move forward on the path to healing. One of the first steps in dealing with fear and anxiety is to recognize when these emotions are present.

By acknowledging and accepting these feelings, individuals can begin to take steps towards managing them effectively.

One way to cope with fear and anxiety is to practice mindfulness and relaxation techniques. This can include deep breathing exercises, meditation, or yoga. These practices can help individuals to stay grounded in the present moment and reduce feelings of overwhelm or panic.

By incorporating these techniques into a daily routine, individuals can begin to cultivate a sense of calm and peace amidst the chaos of dealing with a serious illness.

It is also important for individuals to seek support from loved ones, friends, or a therapist. Talking about fears and anxieties with someone who understands and cares can provide a sense of relief and comfort.

Support groups for individuals with leukemia or lymphoma can also be a valuable resource for connecting with others who are going through similar experiences. Sharing stories and coping strategies with others can help to normalize feelings of fear and anxiety and provide a sense of community and belonging.

In addition to seeking emotional support, taking care of physical health is also crucial in managing fear and anxiety. Regular exercise, a balanced diet, and sufficient sleep can all contribute to overall well-being and reduce feelings of stress.

Engaging in activities that bring joy and relaxation, such as spending time in nature, listening to music, or practicing a hobby, can also help to alleviate fear and anxiety.

Ultimately, it is important for individuals to remember that fear and anxiety are normal responses to a challenging situation.

By acknowledging these emotions, seeking support, and taking care of both emotional and physical health, individuals can begin to navigate through their fears and anxieties and move forward on the journey towards healing and recovery. With time, patience, and self-compassion, it is possible to thrive after leukemia or lymphoma.

Seeking Professional Help

Seeking professional help is a crucial step in the recovery process for individuals who have been diagnosed with leukemia or lymphoma. It is important to remember that you do not have to navigate this journey alone.

There are a variety of healthcare professionals who specialize in treating these types of cancers and can provide you with the support and guidance you need to thrive after your diagnosis.

One of the first professionals you may want to consider seeking help from is an oncologist. An oncologist is a doctor who specializes in the diagnosis and treatment of cancer. They will work with you to develop a personalized treatment plan that is tailored to your specific needs and will monitor your progress throughout your recovery journey.

Your oncologist will also be able to answer any questions you may have about your diagnosis and treatment options, and provide you with the emotional support you need during this challenging time.

In addition to an oncologist, you may also benefit from working with a psychologist or therapist who specializes in working with cancer patients. Dealing with a cancer diagnosis can be overwhelming and may lead to feelings of anxiety, depression, or fear. A mental health professional can provide you with coping strategies and support to help you navigate these emotions and improve your overall well-being. They can also help you develop a positive mindset and cultivate a sense of resilience as you work towards recovery.

Another professional you may want to consider seeking help from is a nutritionist or dietitian. Eating a healthy and balanced diet is crucial for supporting your body's immune system and overall health during and after cancer treatment.

A nutritionist can help you develop a meal plan that meets your nutritional needs and addresses any side effects of treatment, such as loss of appetite or changes in taste. They can also provide you with tips for managing weight gain or loss, as well as strategies for staying hydrated and maintaining your energy levels.

Lastly, it is important to consider seeking help from a support group or counselor who specializes in working with cancer patients. Connecting with others who are going through a similar experience can provide you with a sense of community and understanding that is invaluable during your recovery journey. A support group can also provide you with a safe space to share your thoughts and feelings, as well as offer practical advice and resources for coping with the challenges of living with leukemia or lymphoma. Remember, seeking professional help is not a sign of weakness, but rather a proactive step towards healing and thriving after your diagnosis.

Building a Support System

One of the most important aspects of recovering from leukemia or lymphoma is building a strong support system. Dealing with a cancer diagnosis can be overwhelming and emotionally draining, which is why having a network of people who can provide emotional support, encouragement, and practical help is crucial. Whether it's family, friends, support groups, or healthcare professionals, having a support system in place can make a world of difference in your healing journey.

Family and friends can be a great source of comfort and reassurance during this challenging time. They can offer a listening ear, help with everyday tasks, and provide emotional support when you need it most.

It's important to communicate your needs to your loved ones so they can offer the support that is most helpful to you. Let them know how they can best assist you and don't be afraid to lean on them when you need a helping hand.

Support groups can also be a valuable resource for individuals battling leukemia or lymphoma. Connecting with others who are going through similar experiences can provide a sense of camaraderie and understanding that can be hard to find elsewhere.

Support groups offer a safe space to share your thoughts and feelings, ask questions, and receive advice from others who have been in your shoes. They can also provide valuable information on coping strategies, treatment options, and resources available to cancer patients.

Healthcare professionals, including doctors, nurses, and therapists, play a crucial role in your recovery process. They can provide medical guidance, emotional support, and practical assistance to help you navigate the challenges of living with leukemia or lymphoma.

Don't hesitate to reach out to your healthcare team whenever you have questions or concerns about your treatment plan or side effects. They are there to help you every step of the way and can offer valuable insights and resources to support your healing journey.

In addition to seeking support from others, it's also important to take care of yourself during this time. Make time for self-care activities that bring you joy and relaxation, such as meditation, exercise, or spending time in nature. Prioritize your physical and emotional well-being by eating a healthy diet, getting enough rest, and managing stress in healthy ways.

Remember that healing is a holistic process that involves taking care of your body, mind, and spirit. By building a strong support system and prioritizing self-care, you can empower yourself to thrive after leukemia or lymphoma and create a roadmap to healing that is sustainable and fulfilling.

How To Recover From Leukemia Or Lymphoma

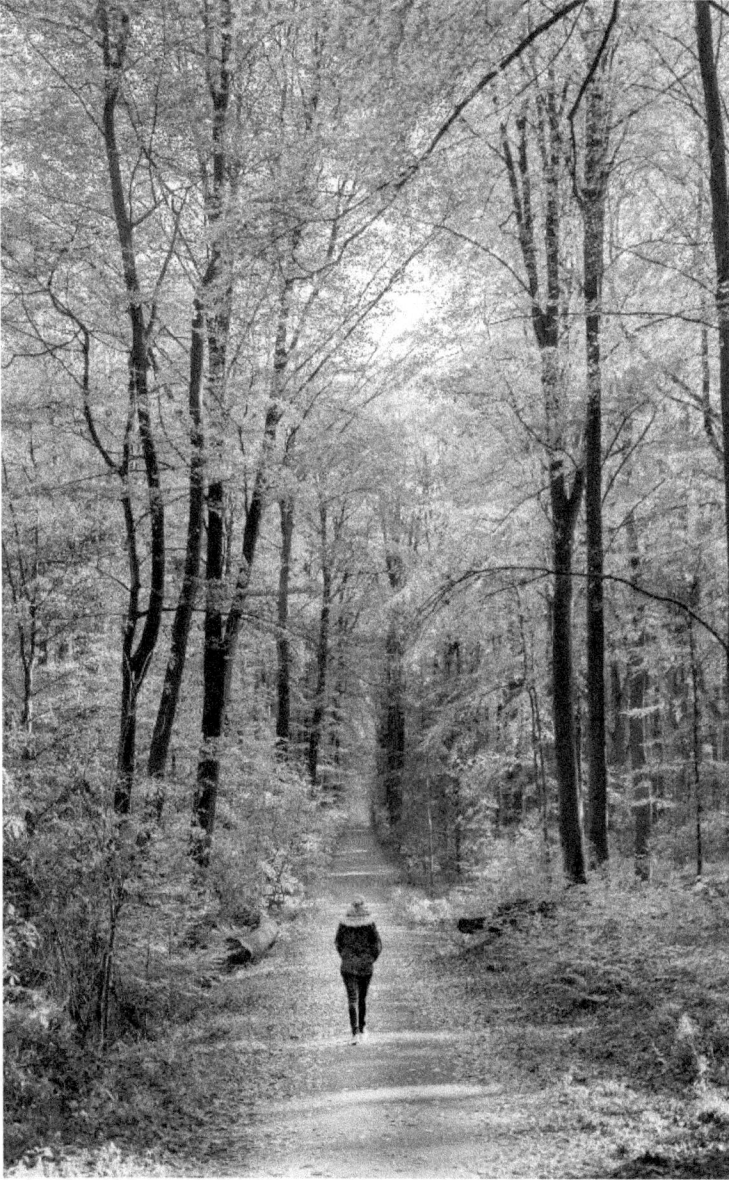

A Roadmap to Healing

Chapter 4

Physical Wellness and Nutrition

Importance of Exercise

Exercise is an essential component of the recovery journey for individuals who have been diagnosed with leukemia or lymphoma. Regular physical activity has been shown to have numerous benefits for cancer survivors, including improved physical strength, reduced fatigue, and enhanced overall well-being. Engaging in exercise can also help to prevent the recurrence of cancer and improve long-term health outcomes.

One of the key benefits of exercise for individuals recovering from leukemia or lymphoma is its ability to improve physical strength and endurance. Cancer treatments such as chemotherapy and radiation therapy can take a toll on the body, leading to muscle weakness and fatigue. By incorporating regular exercise into their routine, survivors can rebuild their strength and stamina, allowing them to better cope with the physical demands of daily life.

In addition to enhancing physical strength, exercise can also help to reduce fatigue and improve overall energy levels for individuals recovering from leukemia or lymphoma. Many cancer survivors experience persistent fatigue as a result of their treatment, which can impact their quality of life and ability to engage in daily activities.

Engaging in regular exercise has been shown to combat fatigue and increase energy levels, helping survivors to feel more alert and active throughout the day.

Furthermore, exercise plays a crucial role in preventing the recurrence of cancer and improving long-term health outcomes for individuals who have been diagnosed with leukemia or lymphoma. Research has shown that regular physical activity can help to reduce the risk of cancer recurrence and improve survival rates for cancer survivors.

By incorporating exercise into their daily routine, individuals can support their body's natural defenses against cancer and promote overall health and well-being.

Overall, the importance of exercise for individuals recovering from leukemia or lymphoma cannot be understated. By engaging in regular physical activity, survivors can improve their physical strength, reduce fatigue, and enhance their overall well-being. Exercise also plays a crucial role in preventing cancer recurrence and improving long-term health outcomes.

As such, it is essential for individuals to prioritize exercise as part of their recovery journey and commit to incorporating regular physical activity into their daily routine.

Healthy Eating Habits

Healthy eating habits are essential for those who have leukemia or lymphoma as they work towards recovering and thriving after their diagnosis. A balanced diet can help boost the immune system, increase energy levels, and support overall well-being.

It is important to focus on incorporating a variety of nutrient-dense foods into your daily meals to support your body's healing process.

One key aspect of healthy eating for those recovering from leukemia or lymphoma is consuming a diet rich in fruits and vegetables. These foods are packed with vitamins, minerals, and antioxidants that can help strengthen the immune system and reduce inflammation in the body. Aim to include a variety of colorful fruits and vegetables in your meals to ensure you are getting a wide range of nutrients.

In addition to fruits and vegetables, it is important to include lean proteins in your diet to support muscle repair and growth. Opt for sources of protein such as lean meats, poultry, fish, eggs, and plant-based proteins like beans and legumes. Protein is essential for healing and recovery, so be sure to include it in each of your meals.

Whole grains are another important component of a healthy diet for those recovering from leukemia or lymphoma. Whole grains provide fiber, vitamins, and minerals that can help support digestion and overall health. Choose whole grain options like brown rice, quinoa, oats, and whole wheat bread to ensure you are getting the most nutritional benefit from your grains.

Lastly, staying hydrated is crucial for those recovering from leukemia or lymphoma. Drinking plenty of water throughout the day can help flush toxins from the body, support digestion, and keep you feeling energized. Aim to drink at least eight glasses of water each day, and consider incorporating herbal teas or infused water for added variety and flavor.

By focusing on incorporating these healthy eating habits into your daily routine, you can support your body's healing process and thrive after leukemia or lymphoma.

Supplements and Vitamins

Supplements and vitamins play a crucial role in the recovery process for individuals who have been diagnosed with leukemia or lymphoma. These essential nutrients can help support the immune system, boost energy levels, and aid in overall healing. It is important for patients to work closely with their healthcare team to determine which supplements and vitamins are best suited for their individual needs.

One of the key supplements that can benefit those recovering from leukemia or lymphoma is vitamin D. Studies have shown that vitamin D plays a vital role in immune function and can help reduce inflammation in the body. Additionally, vitamin D has been linked to lower rates of cancer recurrence in some studies, making it a valuable supplement for individuals post-treatment.

Another important supplement to consider is omega-3 fatty acids, which are known for their anti-inflammatory properties. Omega-3s can help reduce inflammation in the body, improve heart health, and support overall well-being. Incorporating foods rich in omega-3s, such as fatty fish, flaxseeds, and walnuts, or taking a high-quality fish oil supplement can be beneficial for individuals recovering from leukemia or lymphoma.

In addition to specific supplements, ensuring a well-rounded diet that includes a variety of vitamins and minerals is essential for recovery. Foods rich in antioxidants, such as fruits, vegetables, and whole grains, can help support the body's natural defenses and promote healing.

It may also be beneficial to work with a registered dietitian to develop a personalized nutrition plan that meets individual needs and preferences.

Overall, incorporating supplements and vitamins into a comprehensive recovery plan can help individuals thrive after leukemia or lymphoma. By working closely with healthcare providers and focusing on a nutrient-dense diet, individuals can support their immune system, improve energy levels, and enhance overall well-being during the recovery process. Remember, it is important to consult with a healthcare provider before starting any new supplement regimen to ensure safety and effectiveness.

Holistic Healing Practices

Holistic healing practices are becoming increasingly popular among individuals who have been diagnosed with leukemia or lymphoma. These practices focus on treating the whole person, including the mind, body, and spirit, rather than just the disease itself. By incorporating holistic healing practices into your treatment plan, you can enhance your overall well-being and improve your chances of recovery.

One key aspect of holistic healing practices is nutrition. Eating a diet rich in fruits, vegetables, whole grains, and lean proteins can help boost your immune system and support your body's natural healing processes. Avoiding processed foods, sugar, and unhealthy fats can also help reduce inflammation and improve your overall health. Additionally, staying hydrated and maintaining a healthy weight can further support your body's ability to fight off cancer cells.

Another important component of holistic healing practices is exercise. Regular physical activity can help strengthen your body, improve your mood, and reduce stress. Engaging in activities such as yoga, walking, swimming, or tai chi can also help improve your flexibility, balance, and coordination. Finding an exercise routine that works for you and sticking to it can have a positive impact on your physical and emotional well-being.

In addition to nutrition and exercise, holistic healing practices often include stress management techniques such as meditation, deep breathing exercises, and mindfulness practices. These techniques can help calm your mind, reduce anxiety, and improve your overall sense of well-being.

By incorporating stress management techniques into your daily routine, you can better cope with the emotional challenges of living with leukemia or lymphoma and improve your quality of life.

Overall, holistic healing practices offer a comprehensive approach to healing that can complement traditional medical treatments for leukemia and lymphoma. By focusing on treating the whole person – mind, body, and spirit – you can enhance your overall well-being and improve your chances of recovery. Whether you choose to incorporate nutrition, exercise, stress management techniques, or all of the above, finding a holistic approach that works for you can help you thrive after leukemia and lymphoma.

How To Recover From Leukemia Or Lymphoma

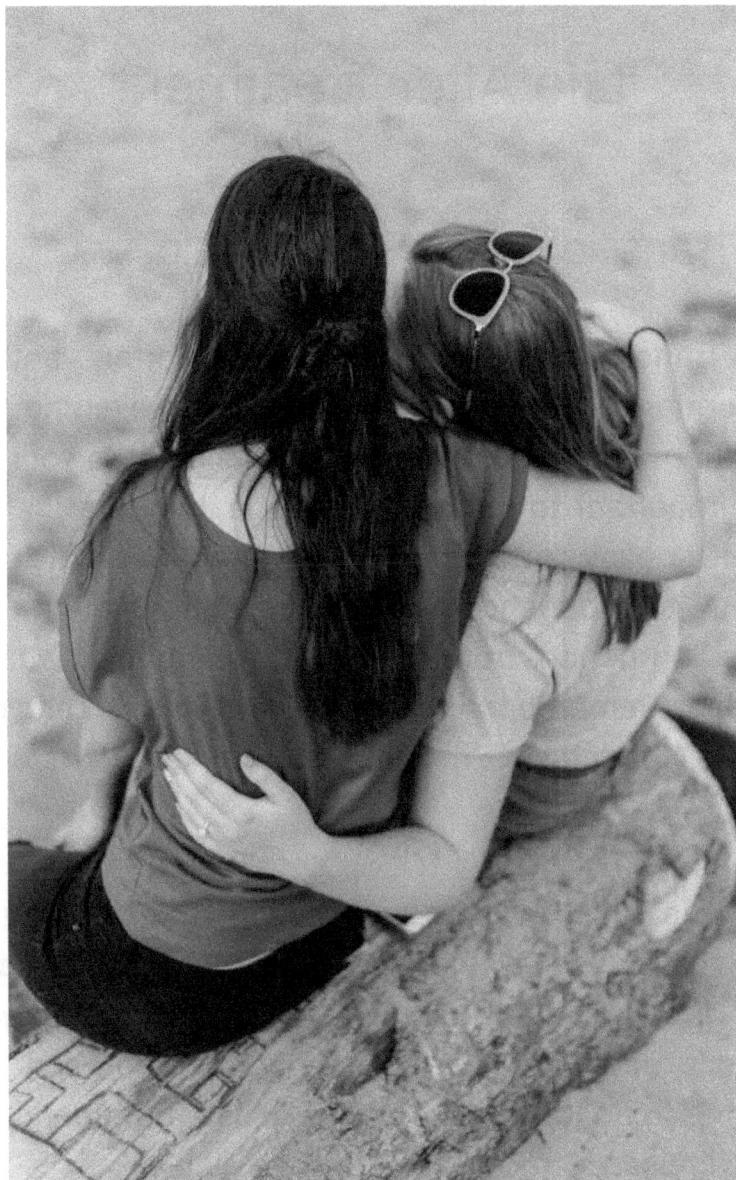

A Roadmap to Healing

Chapter 5

Life After Treatment

Transitioning to Survivorship

Transitioning to survivorship after battling leukemia or lymphoma can be both exciting and daunting. As you navigate this new chapter in your life, it is important to remember that healing is a journey, and it is okay to take things one step at a time. It is normal to experience a range of emotions during this transition period, from relief and gratitude to anxiety and fear. Remember to be gentle with yourself and give yourself permission to feel whatever emotions come up.

One of the key aspects of transitioning to survivorship is developing a new sense of normalcy. Your life may have revolved around treatment and doctor's appointments for so long that it can feel strange to no longer have those constant reminders of your illness.

It is important to find ways to establish a new routine that supports your physical, emotional, and spiritual well-being. This may involve incorporating healthy habits such as regular exercise, nutritious eating, mindfulness practices, and connecting with loved ones.

Another important aspect of transitioning to survivorship is addressing any lingering physical or emotional challenges that may persist after treatment. It is common for survivors to experience side effects from their treatment, such as fatigue, neuropathy, or anxiety.

It is crucial to communicate openly with your healthcare team about any symptoms you may be experiencing so that they can provide you with the necessary support and resources to help you manage these challenges.

In addition to addressing physical and emotional challenges, it is also important to focus on rebuilding your life after leukemia or lymphoma. This may involve setting new goals for yourself, whether they be related to your career, relationships, or personal growth.

Remember that you have overcome incredible challenges and that you have the strength and resilience to create a life that is meaningful and fulfilling for you.

Lastly, remember that transitioning to survivorship is a process that takes time. Be patient with yourself as you adjust to this new phase of life. Surround yourself with a supportive community of friends, family, and healthcare providers who can help you navigate this transition with grace and resilience. Remember that you are not alone in this journey, and that there are resources and support available to help you thrive after leukemia or lymphoma.

Monitoring and Follow-Up Care

Monitoring and follow-up care are crucial components of the recovery process for individuals who have been diagnosed with leukemia or lymphoma. After completing treatment, it is essential to continue with regular check-ups and monitoring to ensure that the cancer does not return. These follow-up appointments allow healthcare providers to closely monitor your health and address any potential concerns that may arise.

' During these follow-up appointments, your healthcare team will perform various tests and screenings to check for any signs of cancer recurrence. These may include blood tests, imaging studies, and physical exams.

It is important to attend these appointments as scheduled and communicate any symptoms or changes in your health to your healthcare provider promptly. Early detection of cancer recurrence can significantly impact treatment outcomes and overall prognosis.

In addition to monitoring for cancer recurrence, follow-up care also focuses on managing any long-term side effects or complications that may arise as a result of treatment.

Many individuals who have undergone treatment for leukemia or lymphoma may experience ongoing health issues, such as fatigue, neuropathy, or emotional distress. Your healthcare team can provide support and resources to help you manage these side effects and improve your quality of life.

It is also essential to maintain a healthy lifestyle and adhere to any recommended lifestyle modifications to support your recovery and reduce the risk of cancer recurrence. This may include maintaining a balanced diet, engaging in regular physical activity, managing stress, and avoiding tobacco and excessive alcohol consumption. Your healthcare team can provide guidance on how to make these lifestyle changes and support you in achieving your health goals.

Overall, monitoring and follow-up care are essential components of the recovery journey for individuals who have been diagnosed with leukemia or lymphoma. By staying vigilant with your follow-up appointments, communicating openly with your healthcare team, and making healthy lifestyle choices, you can support your recovery and reduce the risk of cancer recurrence.

Remember that you are not alone in this journey, and your healthcare team is here to support you every step of the way towards healing and thriving after leukemia or lymphoma.

Dealing with Survivorship Challenges

Surviving leukemia or lymphoma is a major accomplishment, but it is just the beginning of a new journey. As survivors, you may face a unique set of challenges as you navigate life after cancer. It is important to recognize and address these challenges in order to truly thrive after treatment.

One of the primary survivorship challenges faced by those who have battled leukemia or lymphoma is the physical toll that treatment can take on the body. Chemotherapy, radiation, and other treatments can leave survivors feeling weak, fatigued, and in pain. It is important to work with your healthcare team to develop a plan for managing these physical symptoms and regaining your strength.

In addition to physical challenges, survivors of leukemia and lymphoma may also experience emotional and psychological difficulties. The fear of cancer recurrence, anxiety about the future, and the emotional impact of a cancer diagnosis can all take a toll on mental health.

It is important to seek support from loved ones, mental health professionals, and support groups to help manage these feelings and develop coping strategies.

Another common survivorship challenge is navigating the healthcare system and managing long-term follow-up care. Regular check-ups, screenings, and monitoring are essential for detecting any signs of cancer recurrence early. It is important to work closely with your healthcare team to develop a personalized follow-up plan and stay informed about the latest research and treatment options for leukemia and lymphoma survivors.

Financial challenges can also be a significant burden for leukemia and lymphoma survivors. The cost of treatment, medications, and follow-up care can add up quickly and strain your finances.

It is important to explore resources such as financial assistance programs, insurance coverage, and support from organizations like the Leukemia & Lymphoma Society to help alleviate some of this financial burden.

Overall, dealing with survivorship challenges after leukemia or lymphoma requires a proactive and holistic approach to healing. By addressing physical, emotional, psychological, healthcare, and financial challenges, survivors can create a roadmap to thriving after cancer treatment.

Remember, you are not alone in this journey, and there are resources and support systems available to help you navigate the challenges of survivorship and live a full and healthy life.

Thriving in Your New Normal

Thriving in Your New Normal can be a challenging but rewarding journey for those who have battled leukemia or lymphoma. After undergoing treatment and facing the uncertainties of a serious illness, it is important to focus on healing both physically and emotionally.

The transition from being a patient to a survivor can bring about a range of emotions and adjustments, but it is possible to find a sense of normalcy and even thrive in your new chapter of life.

One key aspect of thriving in your new normal is taking care of your physical health. This includes following your doctor's recommendations for follow-up care, maintaining a healthy diet, and engaging in regular exercise.

These practices can help you regain your strength and energy after treatment and reduce the risk of recurrence. It is important to listen to your body and give yourself the time and space you need to recover fully.

In addition to physical health, emotional well-being is also crucial in thriving after leukemia or lymphoma. Many survivors experience a range of emotions, including fear, anxiety, and depression, as they navigate life after cancer.

Seeking support from loved ones, joining a support group, or speaking with a therapist can help you process these emotions and find ways to cope effectively. It is important to be patient and kind to yourself as you adjust to your new normal and find a sense of balance.

Finding purpose and meaning in your life after leukemia or lymphoma can also contribute to thriving in your new normal. This may involve setting new goals, pursuing hobbies or interests that bring you joy, or giving back to others who are going through similar experiences. By focusing on what matters most to you and finding ways to live a fulfilling life, you can create a sense of purpose that gives you strength and resilience in the face of challenges.

Ultimately, thriving in your new normal is a personal journey that requires self-reflection, patience, and resilience. By taking care of your physical and emotional well-being, seeking support when needed, and finding purpose and meaning in your life, you can embrace your survivorship and live a fulfilling and meaningful life after leukemia or lymphoma. Remember that you are not alone on this journey, and there are resources and people who can support you every step of the way.

How To Recover From Leukemia Or Lymphoma

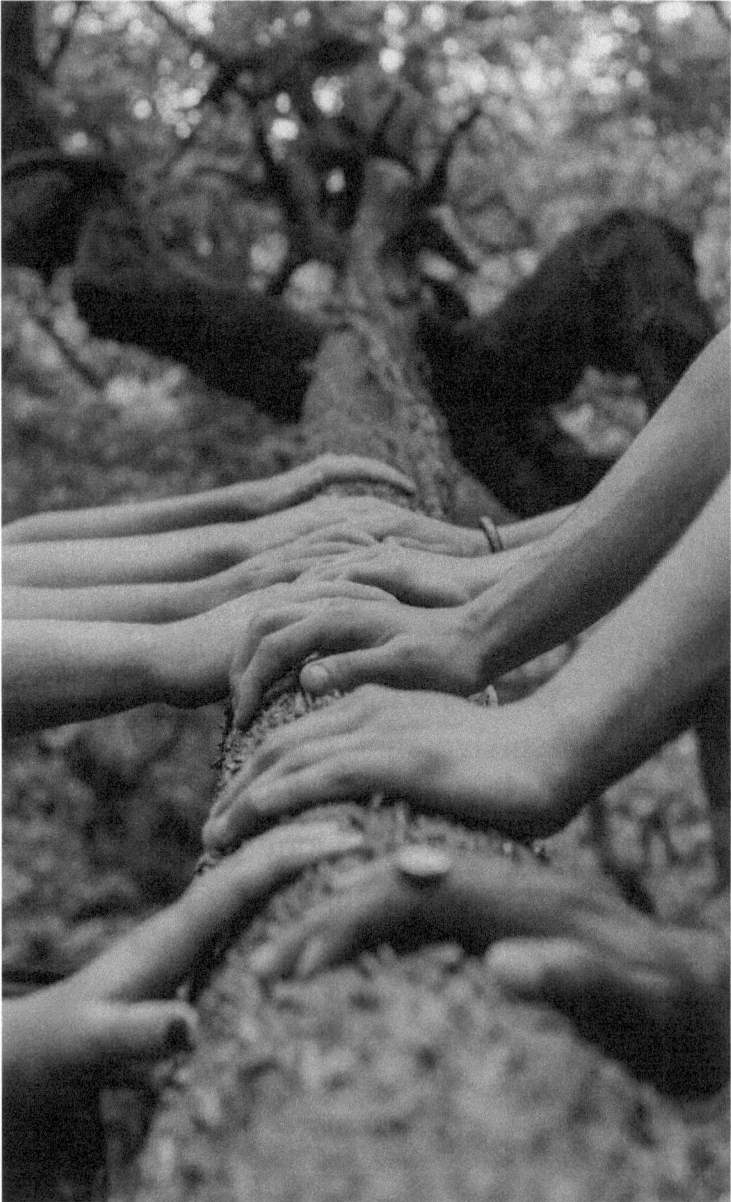

Chapter 6

Resources and Support Networks

Support Groups and Organizations

Support Groups and Organizations play a crucial role in the recovery journey of individuals who have been diagnosed with leukemia or lymphoma. These groups provide a safe and supportive space for patients to share their experiences, fears, and triumphs with others who truly understand what they are going through. By connecting with others who are facing similar challenges, patients can find comfort, strength, and hope in knowing that they are not alone in their battle against cancer.

One of the most well-known organizations that provide support to leukemia and lymphoma patients is the Leukemia & Lymphoma Society (LLS). LLS offers a wide range of resources, including educational materials, support groups, and financial assistance programs to help patients navigate their cancer journey.

By connecting with LLS, patients can access valuable information, connect with other survivors, and find the support they need to thrive after their diagnosis.

In addition to LLS, there are numerous other support groups and organizations that cater to the specific needs of leukemia and lymphoma patients. These groups offer a variety of services, including online forums, in-person support groups, counseling services, and educational workshops.

By participating in these programs, patients can gain valuable insights, tools, and strategies to help them cope with the physical, emotional, and psychological challenges of cancer treatment.

Support groups and organizations also play a vital role in advocating for the needs of leukemia and lymphoma patients. By raising awareness about the unique challenges faced by cancer survivors, these groups help to promote policies and programs that support the health and well-being of patients.

Through their advocacy efforts, support groups and organizations help to ensure that patients have access to quality care, affordable treatment options, and a supportive community to help them on their road to recovery.

In conclusion, support groups and organizations are an invaluable resource for individuals who have been diagnosed with leukemia or lymphoma. By connecting with others who understand their struggles, patients can find comfort, strength, and hope as they navigate their cancer journey.

Through these groups, patients can access a wealth of resources, support, and advocacy to help them thrive after their diagnosis. If you or a loved one is facing leukemia or lymphoma, consider reaching out to a support group or organization to find the help and support you need to heal and thrive.

Financial Assistance Programs

For individuals battling leukemia or lymphoma, the financial burden of treatment can be overwhelming. In this chapter, we will explore various financial assistance programs that are available to help alleviate some of the financial stress that comes with a cancer diagnosis.

These programs can provide much-needed support to help cover medical expenses, transportation costs, and other financial burdens that may arise during treatment.

One important financial assistance program to consider is the Patient Advocate Foundation. This organization offers financial assistance to cancer patients who are struggling to cover the cost of their treatment.

They can help with a variety of expenses, including co-pays, deductibles, and medication costs. Additionally, they offer support services to help patients navigate the complex healthcare system and advocate for their rights as a patient.

Another valuable resource for financial assistance is the Leukemia & Lymphoma Society. This organization provides financial assistance to individuals with blood cancer who are in need of help covering the cost of their treatment. They offer grants to help with medical expenses, transportation costs, and other financial burdens that may arise during treatment.

Additionally, they provide educational resources and support services to help patients and their families cope with the emotional and financial challenges of a cancer diagnosis.

In addition to these national organizations, there are also many local and regional financial assistance programs available to help individuals with leukemia or lymphoma. These programs may offer assistance with transportation costs, lodging expenses, and other practical needs that may arise during treatment. It is important to research and explore all available resources to ensure that you are taking advantage of all the financial assistance programs that are available to you.

Overall, navigating the financial aspects of cancer treatment can be challenging, but it is important to remember that there are resources available to help. By exploring financial assistance programs such as the Patient Advocate Foundation and the Leukemia & Lymphoma Society, as well as local and regional programs, individuals with leukemia or lymphoma can alleviate some of the financial burden that comes with a cancer diagnosis.

Remember, you are not alone in this journey, and there are resources and support available to help you thrive after leukemia or lymphoma.

Educational Materials and Workshops

One of the key components of recovering from leukemia or lymphoma is education. Understanding your diagnosis, treatment options, and how to care for yourself during and after treatment is crucial for your healing journey. That's why we provide a variety of educational materials and workshops to help you navigate this challenging time.

Our educational materials cover a wide range of topics, including the basics of leukemia and lymphoma, different types of treatments available, managing side effects, and tips for self-care. These resources are designed to empower you with knowledge so you can make informed decisions about your health and well-being. From pamphlets and brochures to online resources and videos, we offer a variety of formats to suit your learning style.

In addition to educational materials, we also offer workshops led by healthcare professionals and experts in the field. These workshops cover a range of topics, from nutrition and exercise to stress management and emotional well-being. By participating in these workshops, you can gain practical skills and strategies to support your recovery and overall health.

Our workshops are interactive and provide a supportive environment where you can connect with others who are also on the road to healing. This sense of community can be incredibly powerful and can help you feel less alone during this challenging time.

Whether you attend in-person workshops at our facility or participate in virtual workshops online, you'll have the opportunity to learn, grow, and heal alongside others who understand what you're going through.

Overall, our educational materials and workshops are designed to empower you with the knowledge and skills you need to thrive after leukemia or lymphoma. By taking advantage of these resources, you can become an active participant in your healing journey and set yourself up for a brighter, healthier future. Remember, you are not alone in this journey – we are here to support you every step of the way.

Connecting with Other Survivors

Connecting with other survivors can be an incredibly powerful and healing experience for those who have gone through the difficult journey of leukemia or lymphoma. Sharing your stories, struggles, and triumphs with others who have faced similar challenges can provide a sense of validation and understanding that is hard to find elsewhere.

By connecting with other survivors, you can build a support system that can help you navigate the ups and downs of recovery and provide a sense of community that is essential for healing.

One way to connect with other survivors is through support groups specifically for those who have been diagnosed with leukemia or lymphoma. These groups provide a safe space for individuals to share their experiences, ask questions, and offer support to one another. Being able to talk to others who truly understand what you are going through can be incredibly comforting and can help you feel less alone in your journey.

In addition to support groups, online forums and social media platforms can be great ways to connect with other survivors from all over the world. These platforms allow you to share your story, ask for advice, and offer support to others who are going through similar experiences. By connecting with other survivors online, you can expand your support network and gain valuable insights and perspectives from people who have been in your shoes.

Attending survivorship events and conferences can also be a great way to connect with other survivors in person. These events often feature workshops, panel discussions, and networking opportunities that can help you build relationships with other survivors and learn more about the latest developments in survivorship care. By attending these events, you can gain new insights, make new connections, and feel a sense of camaraderie with others who have overcome similar challenges.

No matter how you choose to connect with other survivors, the important thing is to reach out and make those connections. Building a support network of fellow survivors can provide you with the strength, inspiration, and understanding that you need to thrive after leukemia or lymphoma. Remember, you are not alone in this journey, and there are others out there who are ready and willing to support you every step of the way.

How To Recover From Leukemia Or Lymphoma

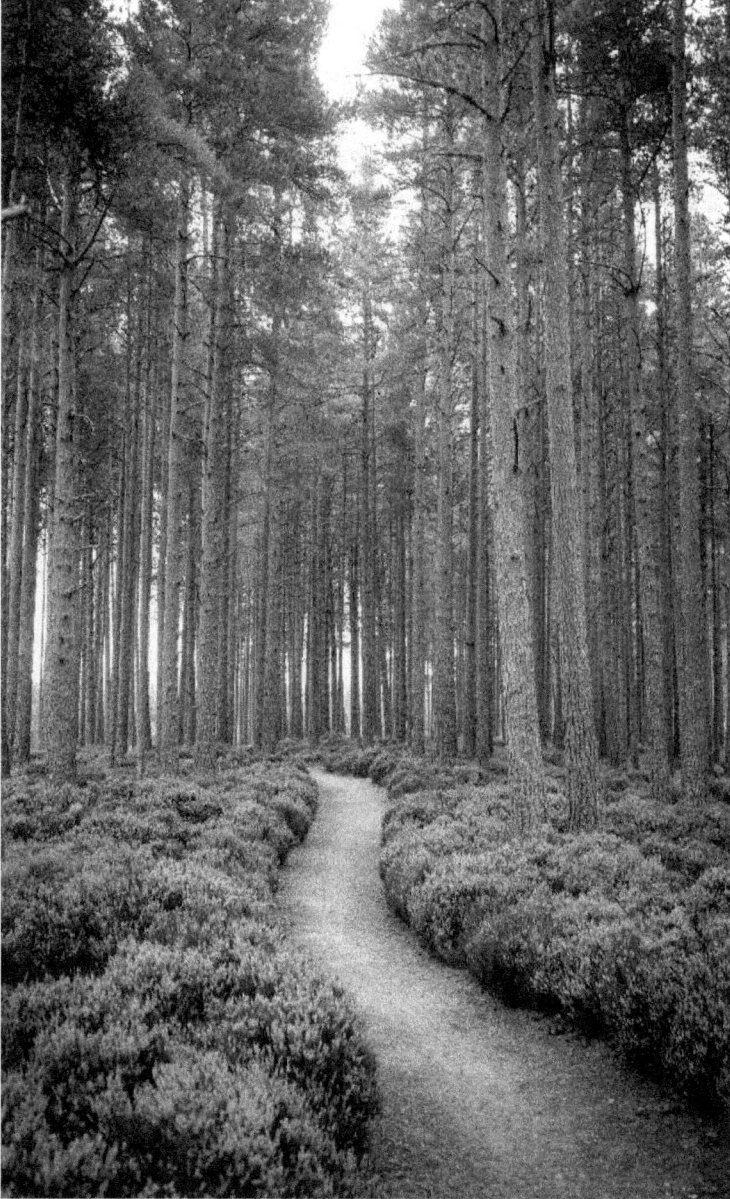

A Roadmap to Healing

Chapter 7

Creating a Personalized Healing Plan

Setting Goals for Recovery

Setting goals for recovery is an essential step in the journey of healing from leukemia or lymphoma. It is important to have a clear vision of what you want to achieve and to set realistic and achievable goals that will help you stay motivated and focused on your recovery.

In this subchapter, we will explore some key strategies for setting goals that will support your physical, emotional, and spiritual well-being as you navigate the challenges of living with these diseases.

One of the first things to consider when setting goals for recovery is to be specific about what you want to achieve. Instead of setting vague goals like "get better," try to break down your objectives into smaller, more manageable tasks.

For example, you might set a goal to walk for 30 minutes a day, or to eat a certain number of servings of fruits and vegetables each day. By being specific about your goals, you can track your progress more effectively and celebrate small victories along the way.

Another important aspect of setting goals for recovery is to make sure they are realistic and achievable. It is important to challenge yourself, but setting goals that are too ambitious can lead to frustration and disappointment. Start by setting small, attainable goals that you can build upon over time.

As you make progress, you can adjust your goals to push yourself a little further, but always remember to be kind to yourself and celebrate your accomplishments, no matter how small they may seem.

In addition to setting physical goals for recovery, it is also important to consider your emotional and spiritual well-being. Setting goals that support your mental health, such as practicing mindfulness or seeking support from a therapist or counselor, can be just as important as physical goals.

Taking care of your emotional and spiritual needs can help you cope with the stress and uncertainty of living with leukemia or lymphoma, and can support your overall well-being as you work towards healing.

Finally, it is important to remember that setting goals for recovery is not a one-time event, but an ongoing process. As you progress in your journey of healing, your goals may need to be adjusted to reflect your changing needs and priorities.

Be flexible and open to reevaluating your goals as needed, and remember that recovery is a journey with ups and downs. By setting realistic, specific, and holistic goals for your recovery, you can stay motivated and focused on the path to healing and thriving after leukemia or lymphoma.

Incorporating Mind-Body Practices

Incorporating mind-body practices is an essential aspect of healing and recovering from leukemia and lymphoma. These practices can help individuals manage stress, reduce anxiety, and improve overall well-being during and after treatment.

By focusing on the connection between the mind and body, individuals can harness the power of their thoughts and emotions to support their physical healing.

One effective mind-body practice that can be incorporated into a healing routine is mindfulness meditation. This practice involves focusing on the present moment and cultivating awareness of one's thoughts, feelings, and sensations. By practicing mindfulness meditation regularly, individuals can reduce stress levels, improve sleep quality, and enhance overall mental clarity. This can be particularly beneficial for individuals undergoing treatment for leukemia or lymphoma, as it can help them cope with the emotional and physical challenges they may face.

Yoga is another powerful mind-body practice that can support individuals in their recovery from leukemia and lymphoma. Yoga combines physical postures, breathing exercises, and meditation to promote flexibility, strength, and relaxation. By practicing yoga regularly, individuals can improve their physical fitness, reduce pain and discomfort, and enhance their overall sense of well-being.

Additionally, yoga can help individuals connect with their bodies and cultivate a sense of inner peace and resilience as they navigate the challenges of cancer treatment.

Incorporating mind-body practices such as guided imagery and visualization can also be beneficial for individuals recovering from leukemia and lymphoma. These practices involve using mental imagery to create positive, healing experiences in the mind. By visualizing themselves healthy, strong, and free from disease, individuals can harness the power of their imagination to support their physical healing. Guided imagery and visualization can help individuals cultivate a sense of hope, empowerment, and optimism as they work towards recovery.

Overall, incorporating mind-body practices into a healing routine can support individuals in their recovery from leukemia and lymphoma. By exploring practices such as mindfulness meditation, yoga, guided imagery, and visualization, individuals can tap into the mind-body connection to promote healing, reduce stress, and enhance overall well-being.

These practices can be powerful tools for individuals navigating the challenges of cancer treatment and can help them thrive on their journey to healing.

Tracking Your Progress

Tracking your progress is an essential part of your journey to recovery from leukemia or lymphoma. By keeping track of your symptoms, treatments, and overall well-being, you can better understand how your body is responding to the disease and treatment. This information can help you and your healthcare team make informed decisions about your care and make adjustments as needed.

One way to track your progress is to keep a journal or diary. Write down any symptoms you are experiencing, as well as how you are feeling physically and emotionally. Note any side effects from treatment, changes in appetite or energy levels, and any other important details. This information can provide valuable insights into patterns and trends in your health that can help guide your treatment plan.

In addition to keeping a journal, it can be helpful to track specific markers of your health, such as your white blood cell count, platelet count, and hemoglobin levels. By monitoring these markers regularly, you can see how they are responding to treatment and identify any trends that may require intervention. Your healthcare team can help you understand the significance of these markers and how to interpret the results.

Another important aspect of tracking your progress is setting goals for yourself. Whether it's improving your energy levels, managing side effects better, or reaching a specific milestone in your treatment plan, setting goals can help keep you motivated and focused on your recovery. Make sure your goals are realistic and achievable, and celebrate your successes along the way.

Finally, don't be afraid to ask for help when tracking your progress. Your healthcare team, friends, and family members can provide valuable support and guidance as you navigate the ups and downs of recovery.

By working together and staying proactive in monitoring your health, you can empower yourself to thrive after leukemia or lymphoma. Remember, every small step forward is a victory on your road to healing.

Adjusting Your Plan as Needed.

Adjusting Your Plan as Needed

Receiving a diagnosis of leukemia or lymphoma can be overwhelming and life-changing. As you begin your journey towards healing and recovery, it is important to remember that your treatment plan may need to be adjusted along the way. Each person's body responds differently to treatment, and it is essential to listen to your body and communicate openly with your healthcare team about any changes or concerns you may have.

One of the key components of thriving after leukemia or lymphoma is being flexible and willing to make changes to your treatment plan as needed. Your healthcare team will monitor your progress closely and may recommend adjustments to your medications, therapies, or lifestyle habits based on your response to treatment.

It is important to trust their expertise and be open to trying new approaches that may improve your overall well-being.

It is also important to be proactive in advocating for yourself and seeking out additional support or resources if you feel that your current treatment plan is not meeting your needs. Don't be afraid to ask questions, express your concerns, or seek a second opinion if necessary. Remember, you are the expert on your own body, and it is crucial to be an active participant in your own healing journey.

In addition to making adjustments to your treatment plan, it is also important to focus on self-care and maintaining a positive mindset throughout your recovery process. Surround yourself with supportive friends and family members, engage in activities that bring you joy and relaxation, and prioritize your physical and emotional well-being. Remember that healing is a holistic process, and taking care of yourself on all levels is essential for a successful recovery.

By staying flexible, advocating for yourself, and prioritizing self-care, you can navigate the challenges of adjusting your treatment plan as needed and continue on the path towards healing and thriving after leukemia or lymphoma. Remember, you are not alone in this journey, and there are many resources and support systems available to help you along the way. Stay strong, stay positive, and never lose hope for a brighter, healthier future ahead.

Author Notes & Acknowledgments

First and foremost, I would like to express my deepest gratitude to the people who inspired and supported me throughout the journey of writing this book. This project would not have been possible without their unwavering belief in me and their invaluable contributions.

To my wife, thank you for your constant encouragement and understanding. Your love and support have been my anchor during the challenging times of researching and writing this book. Your belief in my ability to make a difference in people's lives has been my driving force.

I would also like to disclose that this book contains some renewed artificial intelligence-generated content. I really appreciate very recent technological innovation by outstanding scientists and of course our reader's understanding.

Lastly, I want to express my deepest gratitude to the readers of this book. I sincerely hope the strategies and methods outlined within these pages will provide you with the knowledge and tools needed to truly make your life much better. Your commitment to seeking any good solutions and willingness to explore multiple methods is commendable.

Author Bio

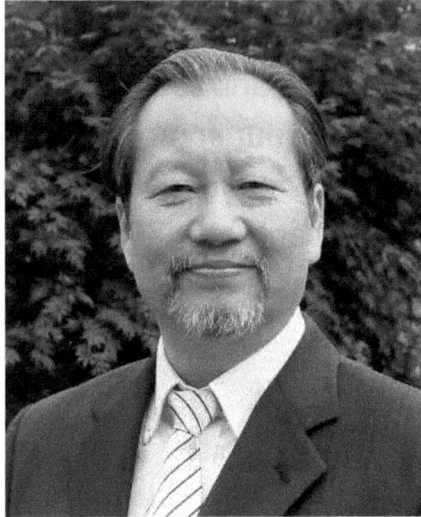

Johnson Wu earned his MD in 1982. With over 40 years of clinical experience, he has worked in hospitals in Zhejiang and Shanghai, China, as well as the Royal Marsden Hospital (part of Imperial College) in London, UK.

Upon the recommendation of Sir Aaron Klug, the president of The Royal Society and a Nobel Prize winner in Chemistry, Dr. Wu was honorably awarded a British Royal Society Fellowship. He has published medical books and articles in seven countries and currently practices medicine in Canada.

www.ingramcontent.com/pod-product-compliance
Lightning Source LLC
Chambersburg PA
CBHW060256030426

42335CB00014B/1717